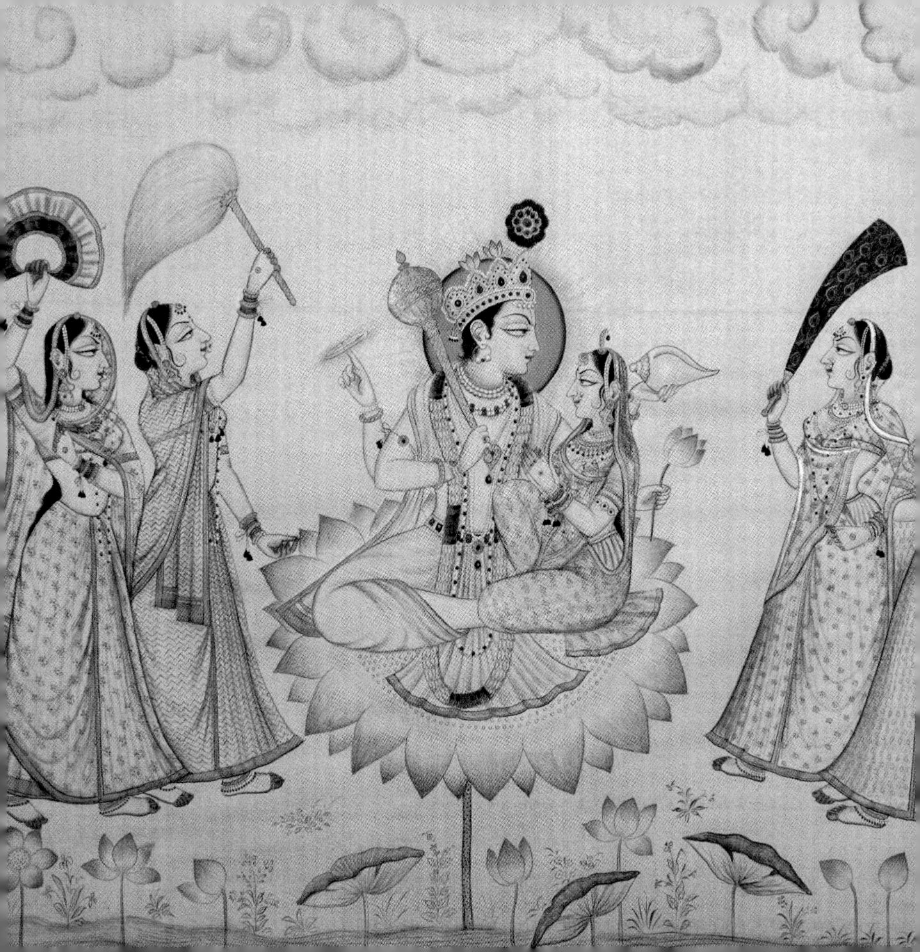

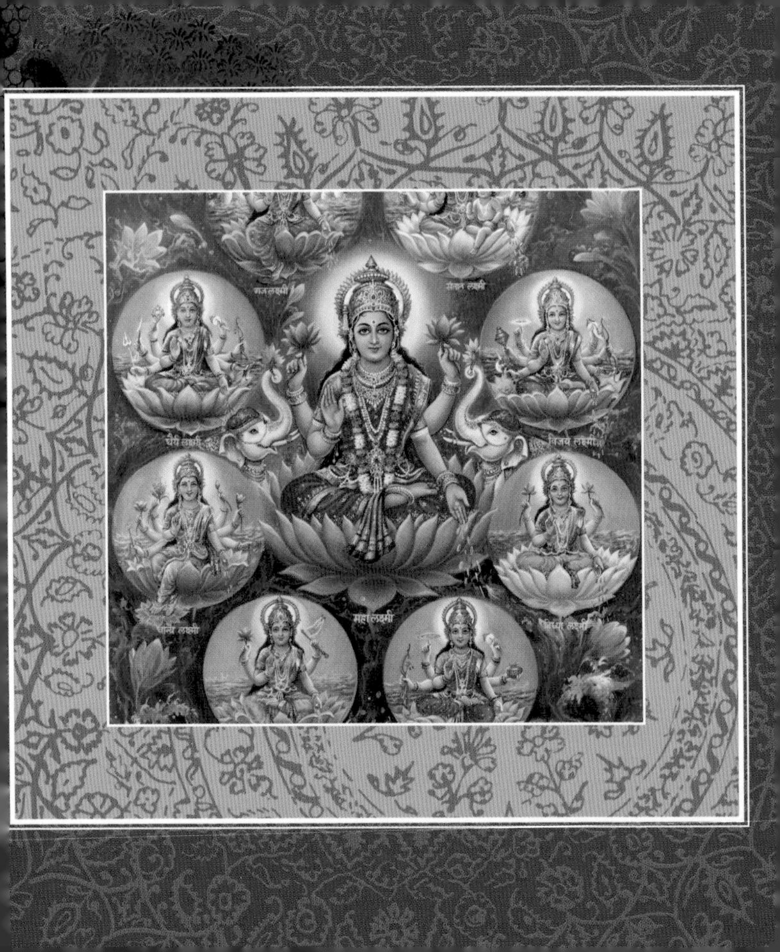

विजय लक्ष्मी
महा लक्ष्मी

an electrical wire properly connected can produce light, so when we are properly oriented, we may vibrate the name of God and bring light to the world through divine sound.

Here we have to differentiate the concept of vibrating and hearing the divine name and its effects upon the sincere spiritual aspirant from many of the popular sound inventions offered today for balancing our brain waves. Sometimes these inventions are advertised as being capable of producing the same effect that previously took lifetimes of dedication and sacrifice to achieve, in a relatively short period of time—say, 30 minutes. Certain synchronized sound patterns, it may be demonstrated, produce a similar effect upon the brain as that which is observed by researchers who study those who submit themselves to experimentation during meditation. Fine. But it is a long jump from there to the "30 minute" ads. We must remember that because one person's brain functions similarly to another's, that says nothing about the similarity of their hearts. Such experiments may inadvertently support the reductionist worldview that the spiritual viewpoint repudiates. What is more, it is easy to understand how two opposite sources of stimuli can produce the same physical effect. Tears, for example, can be produced either from emotions of sadness or happiness.

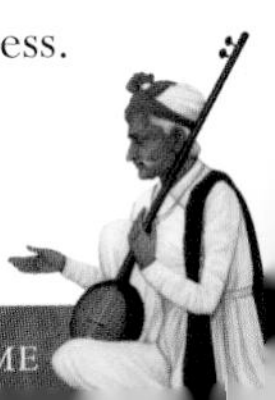

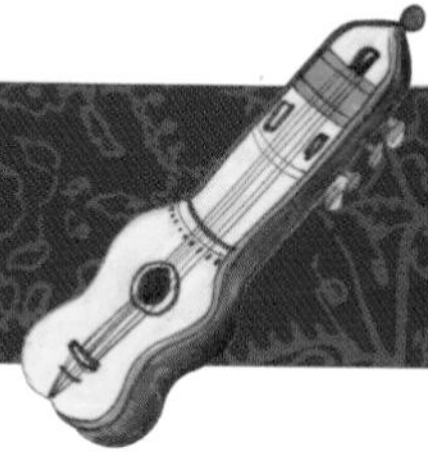

Names as the Path to Devotion

God is more than mundane sound, and the sound that represents God in this world is not something we can manufacture in the recording studio. We may be able to produce many wonderful sounds, even ones that "create," and there is no harm in such experimentation, but the experience of God consciousness is something that will have to descend to us from above. We need only to open our hearts to receive divine sounds.

When discussing the holy name, the Vedic literature—especially the purely devotional texts—mentions many names of God and his energy or *shakti*, the Goddess. It would certainly be questionable if we were to limit the divine to but one name, especially when we ourselves have at least two and usually more. In the Vedas, the many names of God are divided into two sections, primary and secondary. Secondary names are those that describe something about God's attributes in reference to his general presence in the world of *maya,* or illusion. One example

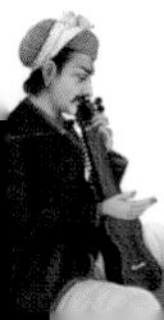

is *Brahman*, which refers to the underlying foundation, undifferentiated consciousness, out of which the mayic world arises. *Paramatma* is another such name that refers to the Oversoul that accompanies the *jivatma*, or finite living being, throughout the material sojourn, acting as witness to all of our karmic deeds. Uttering these names attentively can bring liberation.

Direct names are those that refer to a more intimate concept of God and Goddess as divine beings endowed with personal attributes, and accompanied by innumerable associates in transcendental abodes, such as Radha-Krishna, Sita-Rama, and Lakshmi-Narayana. Those who have accepted in principle that the name of God is sacred relish this latter concept considerably. Such votaries of the holy names are perhaps the best to look to, should we care to explore this principle that, again, is mentioned universally throughout the religious world. That which is mentioned throughout is wholly applied by those engaged exclusively in the practice of chanting the name of God as a means of divine culture.

To this group of votaries, the uttering of the name is more than a means by which to achieve liberation. Although many others do chant primary names of God with a view to achieve liberation, theirs is not the culture of pure devotion per se. Theirs is the culture of knowledge mixed with devotion.

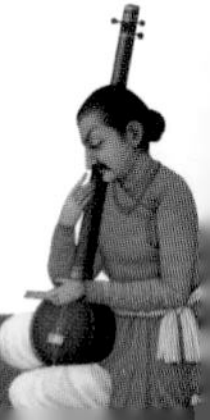

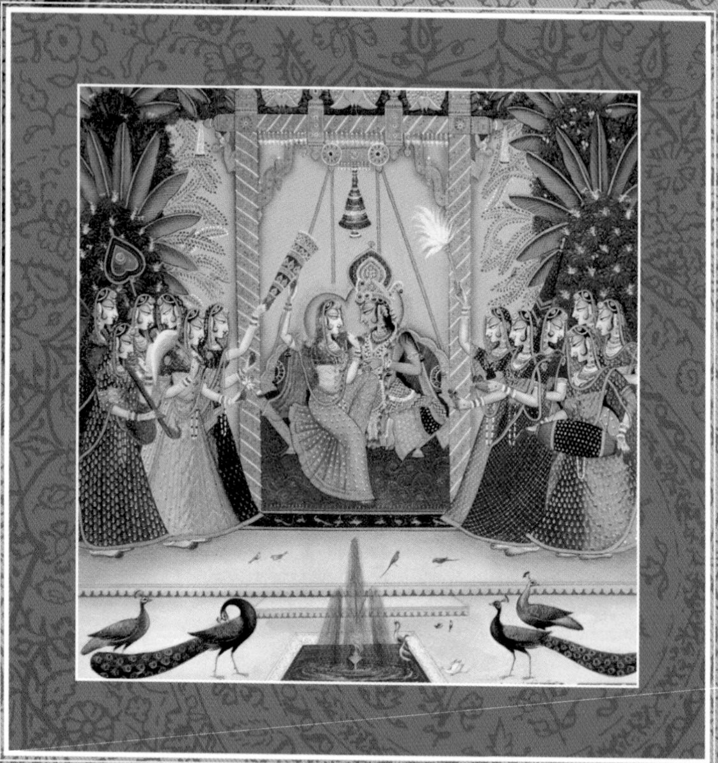

Those that vibrate the names of God in order to achieve liberation, thinking that any name of the divine is equal to any other, may encounter transcendence as a vague experience. It may be like awakening from a deep sleep, having experienced something that is tangible yet indescribable. They agree that the name is not physical sound, maintaining that it is mental and thus within the jurisdiction of illusion. Yet being of the material quality of goodness (*sattva guna*), its incantation has the power to elevate one to the shore of transcendence. Such transcendentalists contend that transcendence is formless and ultimately soundless. Their experience of transcendence, derived from culturing their particular conception of the name is one of a qualityless, varietyless, homogeneous conscious substance, Brahman.

This understanding of transcendence is considered to be elementary by those who maintain that the divine name is a "supramental" sound representation of Godhead. The concept of a supramental name attributes ultimate divinity to the name, which is considered to wholly correspond with the transcendental form of Godhead and a world of transcendental variegatedness. The logic of this transcendental viewpoint, as opposed to the idea of a soundless, formless absolute, may be better appreciated through the following example: as islands arise out of water in the sea from time to time, it may be thought that water is

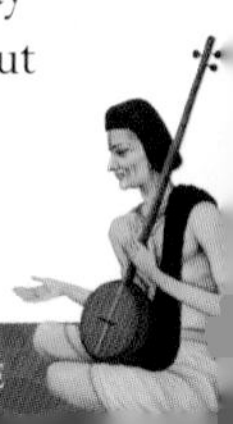

their foundation; similarly, it is true that the world of temporary names and forms arise out of a sea of consciousness, only to disappear in due course. Yet there is also life within the sea. Experiencing the plane of consciousness as varietyless is like describing the ocean as wet—a rather shallow understanding of what makes up the sea. Actually the ocean consists of so many waves, not to mention the world of sea life beneath her surface. As sea life is similar to but not the same as life on land, so the world of consciousness replete with forms and names is different from the world of material names and forms. As everything in the ocean is wet, so too is everything in the conscious world conscious. Thus, within the conception of a supramental name is an invitation to "dive deep" into the world of consciousness.

For those engaged in pure devotion, vibrating the supramental name is both the means and the end of their culture of divinity. Within the pure name, the form, qualities, and pastimes of Godhead are contained. The perfection of the culture of the divine name lies in accessing the spiritual realm and participating in the divine love sports of the Absolute—a very lofty ideal. Liberation from the cycle of birth and death, which is the goal of most transcendentalists, is incidental to those engaged in this culture. It is said that the mere reflection of the pure name of Godhead, rather than the name proper, brings about the

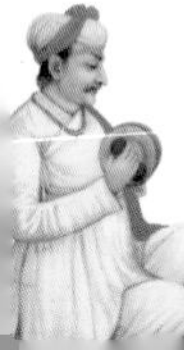

termination of the cycle of birth and death. The practical idea of liberation in which one is progressively freed from all of the painful constituents of our life of bondage, such as lust, anger, greed, envy, and pride, are passed over in the course of approaching only the blossoming of the culture of the holy name. Its flower—*prema*, or love of Godhead—belittles liberation as but the other side of the coin of material exploitation. Enjoyment and renunciation, which produce the effects of karma and liberation, respectively, are both worldly centered. One mentality is to "enjoy" the world of illusion (good luck!) and the other is to flee from it. Both mentalities fall short of a transcendental synthesis of these two principles that govern the mayic world. Transcendence cannot be the polarization of opposites; it must be the synthesis of both thesis and antithesis. Thus, dedication is the

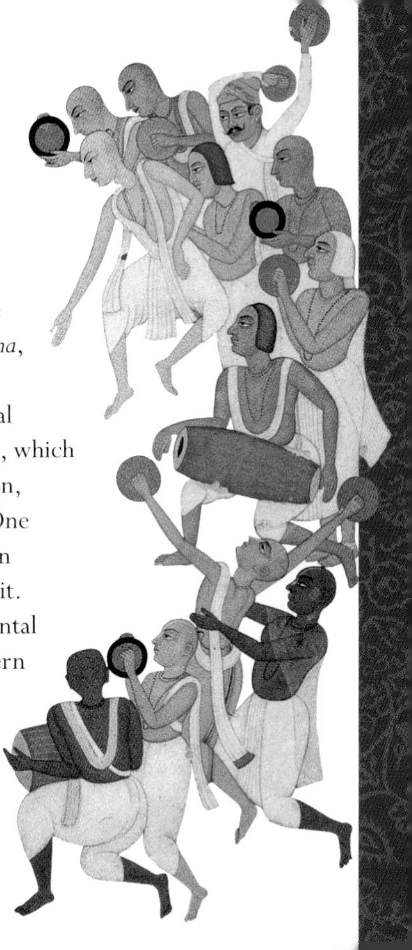

focus of the servants of the divine name, through which exploitation and renunciation are harmonized.

If God is light, as the school of renunciation likes to say, then God is surely sound as well, the two being but the same wave vibrations at different frequencies. But God is more than light and sound as we know them. If there is transcendental light, why not sound? Through the medium of sound, the world comes into being, and through divine sound it can be properly understood. The Vedas and Upanishads are called *shruti*, that which is heard. *Upanishad* in particular means to come closer to hear something confidential. A name is a rather confidential thing to know about the Absolute—a good start. To know the name of the object of our search is the beginning of our finding that truth in a systematic fashion. But it is more than that, because the name of God wholly corresponds with the object of His person.

In the material world of duality, we are troubled by the fact that the names of objects, often given so arbitrarily, do not wholly correspond with the object they seek to describe. The actual sound of a thing, upon being heard, brings us a profound sense of the experience itself. This is so even within the world of duality; how much more so is this the case in a realm where sound and object wholly correspond with one another? The name of God and the sound of God, "OM," carry with them the

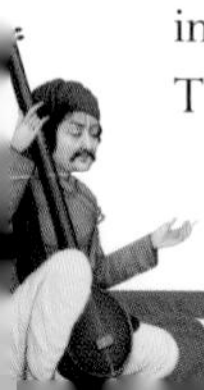

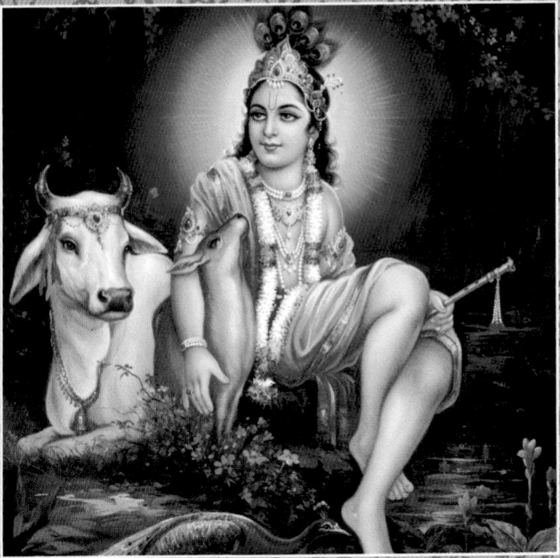

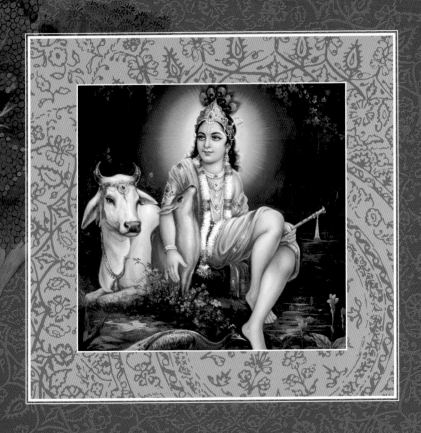

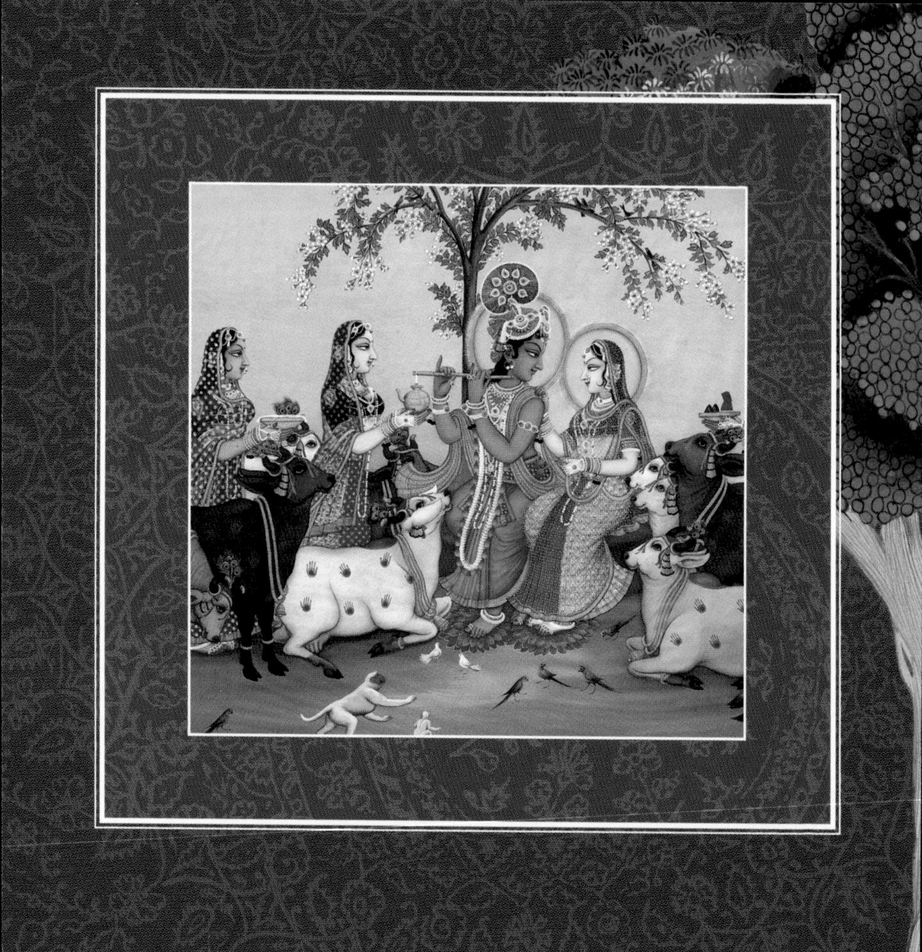

experience of Godhead. And the name more fully than God's sound, for it includes something about the personality of the divine.

The supramental sound of the name of God can be heard and sung only when our dedicating function is directed toward the divine. That such a sound exists will not be possible to understand unless we change the direction of our dedication. We must consider dedication for its own sake if we are to know our highest prospect.

Love, pure love, must be the goal of all existence, and the holy name of God is a "love note" of the divine symphony. It should be allowed to enter our hearts. Actually, if the holy name should desire to descend within our hearts, we cannot keep it out. It is said of the name "Krishna" that it is lucky for us that he is a thief (as the Krishna avatar was known to steal yogurt in divine sport): we have constructed high walls around our hearts, within which we attempt to protect the paltry sense of "I," "me," and "mine" that makes up our egoistic material existence. A thief, however, does not care about high walls.

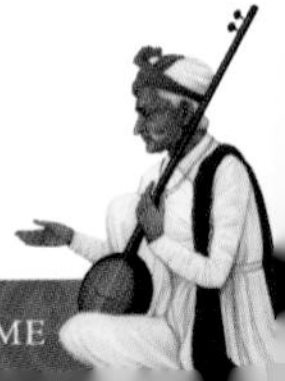

SONGS AND TRANSLATIONS

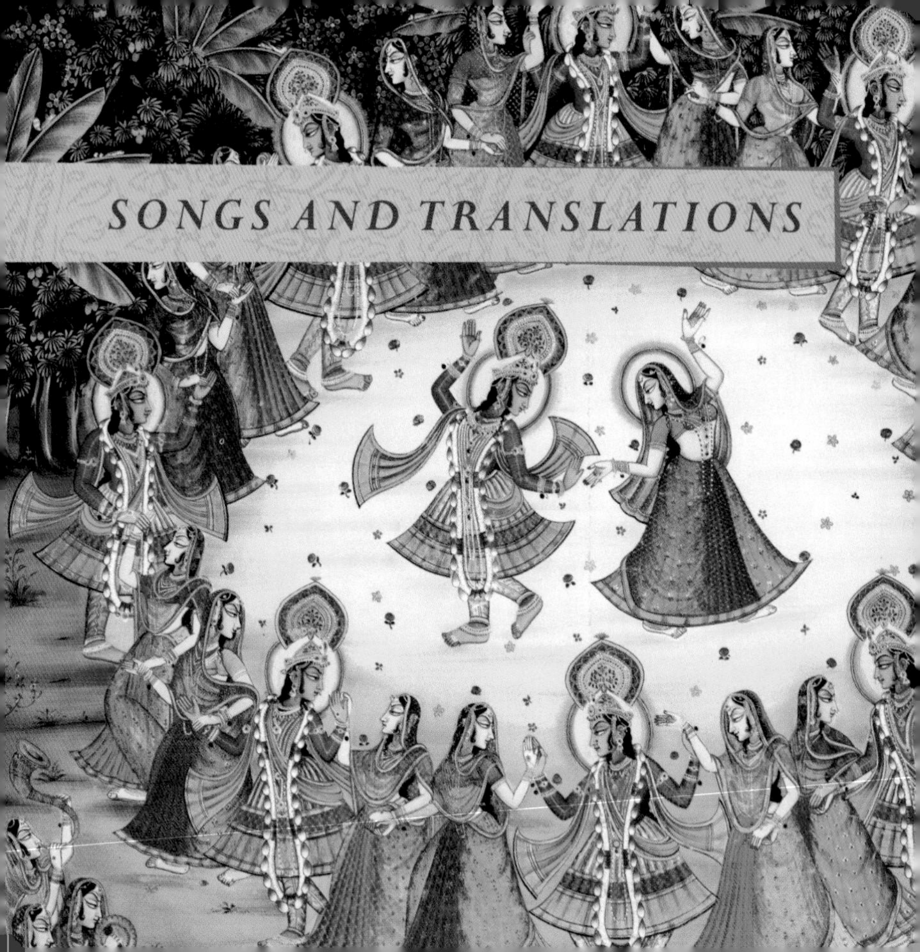

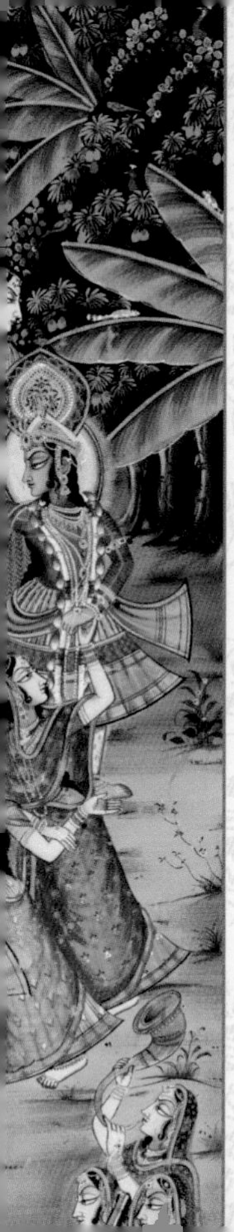

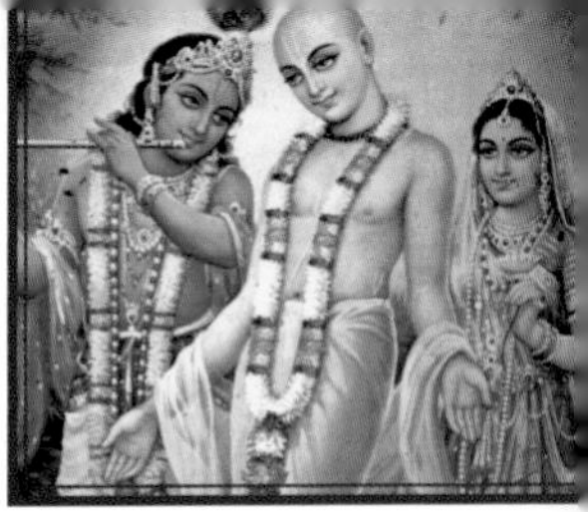

This CD features a selection of songs composed by the bhakti saints of the Gaudiya Vaishnava tradition. Some of the songs are written in Sanskrit, the others in Bengali—a vernacular with close ties to Sanskrit. The songs mostly center on the glorification of the holy names and sacred pastimes of Godhead, of whom Krishna and His divine consort Radha are primary. Although translations are included, understanding the words (which may be difficult without knowledge of the tradition) is not required to reap the benefits of the sacred sound vibrations.

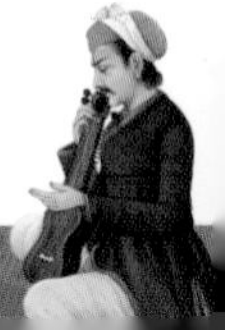

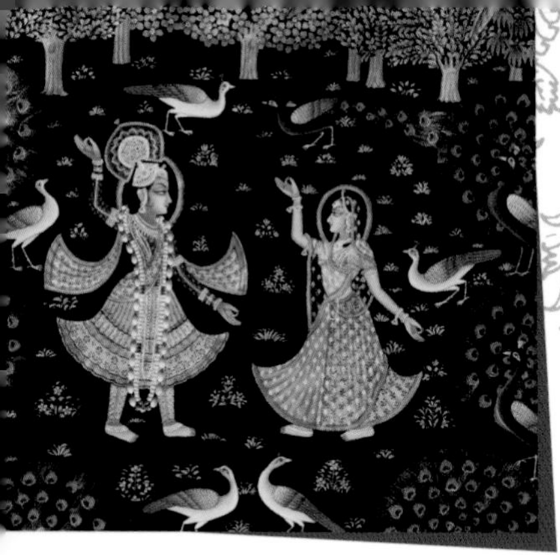

~ Maha Mantra 1 ~

Hare Krishna, Hare Krishna, Krishna Krishna, Hare Hare,
Hare Rama, Hare Rama, Rama Rama, Hare Hare.

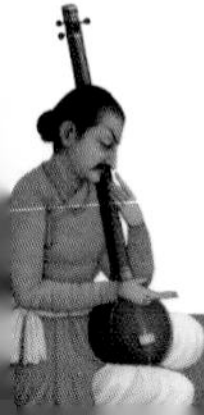

~ Śrī Nāma ~

"The Divine Name"
by Srila Bhaktivinode Thakur

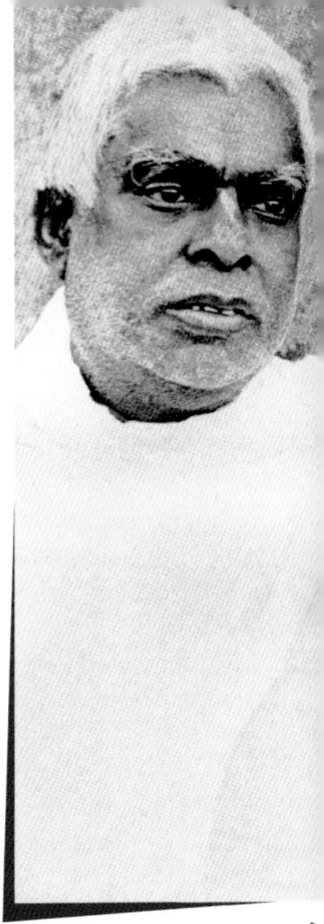

one

gāy gorā madhur sware
hare kṛṣṇa hare kṛṣṇa kṛṣṇa kṛṣṇa hare hare
hare rāma hare rāma rāma rāma hare hare

two

gṛhe thāko, vane thāko, sadā hari bole ḍāko,
sukhe duḥkhe bhulo nāko, vadane hari-nām koro re

three

māyā-jāle baddha hoye, ācho miche kāja loye,
ekhona cetana peye, rādhā mādhava nām bolo re

four

jīvana hoilo śeṣa, nā bhajile hṛṣīkeśa
bhaktivinodopadeśa, ekbār nām-rase māto re

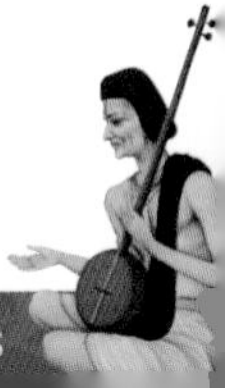

one

Lord Gaurasundar sings the great mantra in a very sweet voice: Hare Krishna, Hare Krishna, Krishna Krishna, Hare Hare, Hare Rama, Hare Rama, Rama Rama, Hare Hare.

two

Whether you are a householder or a renunciate, constantly chant "Hari! Hari!" Do not forget this chanting of the Lord's names, whether you are in a happy condition or a distressful one. Just fill your lips with the harinam.

three

You are bound up in the network of Maya and forced to toil meaninglessly. Now you have understood what this life is meant for, so chant the names of Radha and Madhava.

four

Your life may end at any moment, and you have not served the Lord of the senses, Hrishikesh. Take this advice of Bhaktivinode Thakur: "Just once, relish the nectar of the Holy Name!"

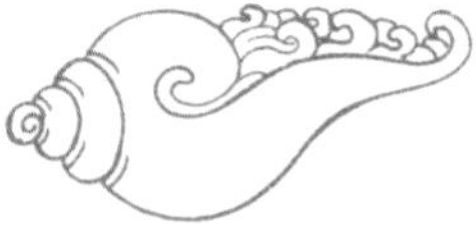

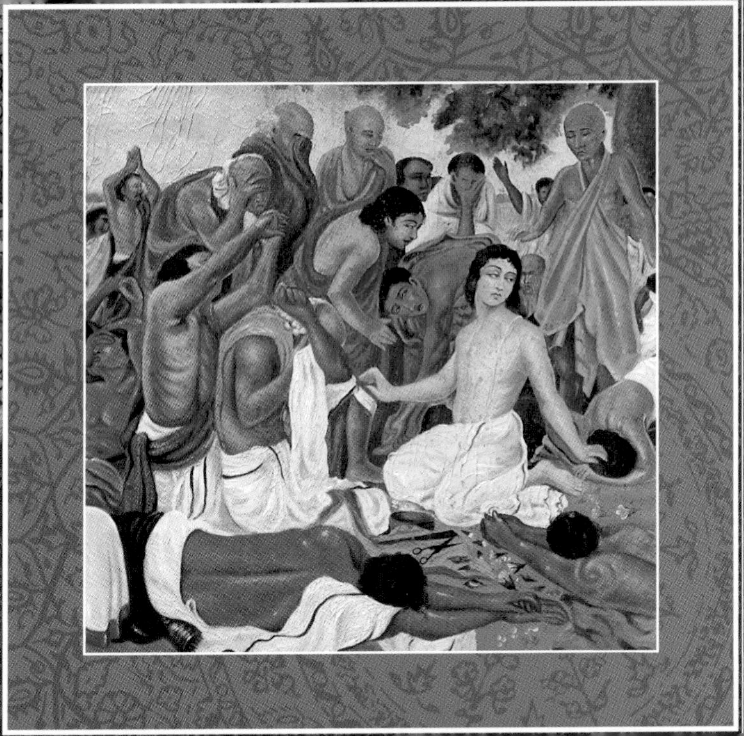

~ Śrī Vraja-dhāma-mahimāmṛta ~

"Glories of Vraja Dham"
by Srila Krishnadas Kaviraj

one

jaya rādhe, jaya kṛṣṇa, jaya vṛndāvan
śrī govinda, gopīnātha, madana-mohan

two

śyama-kunḍa, rādhā-kuṇḍa, giri-govardhan
kālindi jamunā jaya, jaya mahāvan

three

keśī-ghāṭa, vaṁśi-vaṭa, dwādaśa-kānan
jāhā saba īlā koilo śrī-nanda-nandan

four

śrī-nanda-jaśodā jaya, jaya gopa-gaṇ
śrīdāmādi jaya, jaya dhenu-vatsa-gaṇ

five

jaya bṛṣabhānu, jaya kīrtidā sundarī
jaya paurṇamāsī, jaya ābhīra-nāgarī

six

jaya jaya gopīśwara vṛndāvana-mājh
jaya jaya kṛṣṇa-sakhā baṭu dwija-rāj

seven

jaya rāma-ghāta, jaya rohiṇī-nandan
jaya jaya vṛndāvana-bāsī joto jan

eight

jaya dwija-patnī, jaya nāga-kanyā-gaṇ
bhaktite jāhārā pāilo govinda-caraṇ

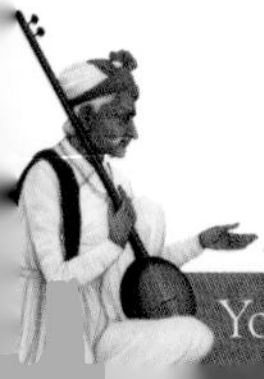

nine

śrī-rasa-maṇḍala jaya, jaya rādhā-śyām
jaya jaya rasa-līlā sarva-manoram

ten

jaya jayojjwala-rasa sarva-rasa-sār
parakīyā-bhāve jāhā brajete pracār

eleven

śrī-jāhnavā-pāda-padma koriyā smaraṇ
dīna kṛṣṇa-dāsa kohe nāma-saṅkīrtan

one

All glories to Radha and Krishna and the transcendental forest of Vrindavan. All glories to the three presiding deities of Vrindavan—Sri Govinda, Gopinath, and Madan Mohan.

two

All glories to Shyama-kund, Radha-kund, Govardhan hill, and the Yamuna river. All glories to the great forest known as Mahavan, where Krishna and Balaram displayed all of Their childhood pastimes.

three

All glories to Keshi-ghat (where Krishna killed the Keshi demon). All glories to the Vamshi-vata tree (where Krishna attracted all the gopis by playing His flute). All glories to the twelve forests of Vraja. At these places, the son of Nanda, Sri Krishna, performed all of His pastimes.

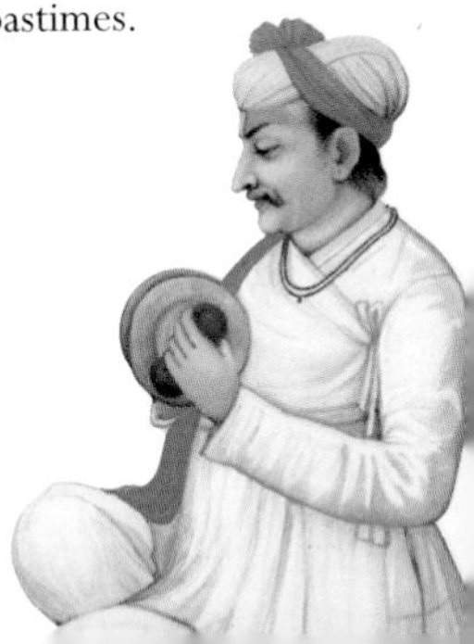

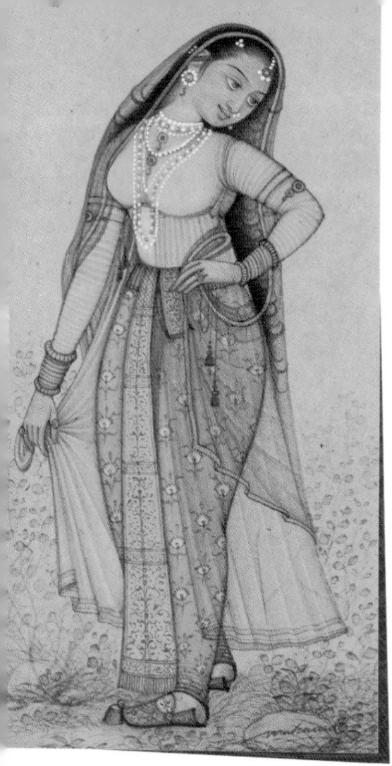

four

All glories to Nanda and Yashoda (Krishna's divine father and mother). All glories to the cowherd boys, headed by Sridam (the older brother of Srimati Radharani and Ananga Manjari). All glories to the cows and calves of Vraja.

five

All glories to Vrishabhanu and the beautiful Kirtida (Radha's divine father and mother). All glories to Paurnamasi (the mother of Sandipani Muni, grandmother of Madhumangal and Nandimukhi). All glories to the young cowherd maidens of Vraja.

six

All glories, all glories to Gopishwar Shiva, who resides in Vrindavan (in order to protect the holy dham). All

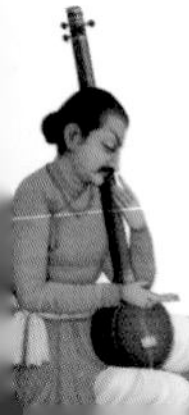

glories to Krishna's funny brahmin friend, Madhumangal.

seven

All glories to Ram-ghat (where Lord Balaram performed his rasa dance). All glories to Lord Balaram, the son of Rohini. All glories, all glories to all of the residents of Vrindavan.

eight

All glories to the wives of the proud Vedic brahmins. All glories to the wives of the Kaliya serpent. Through pure devotion, they all obtained the lotus feet of Lord Govinda.

nine

All glories to the place where the rasa dance of Sri Krishna was performed. All glories to Radha and Shyama. All glories, all glories to the divine rasa dance, which gives the most pleasure to the heart.

ten

All glories to the mellow of conjugal love, which is the essence (sar) of all rasas and is propagated in Vraja by Sri Krishna in the form of the divine parakiya-bhava (paramour love).

eleven

Remembering the lotus feet of Lord Nityananda's consort, Sri Jahnava Devi, Dina Krishna Das sings the sankirtan of the Holy Name.

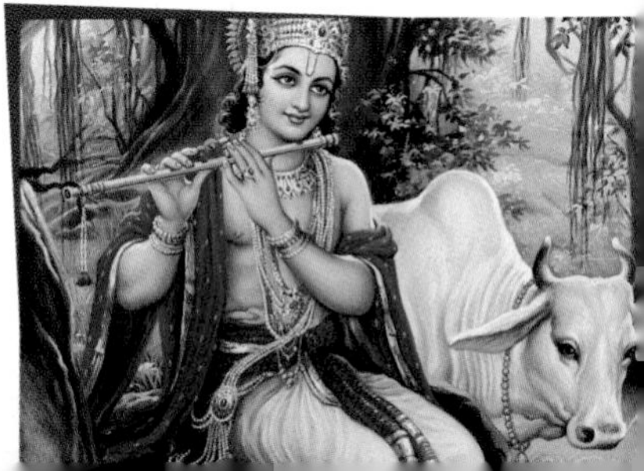

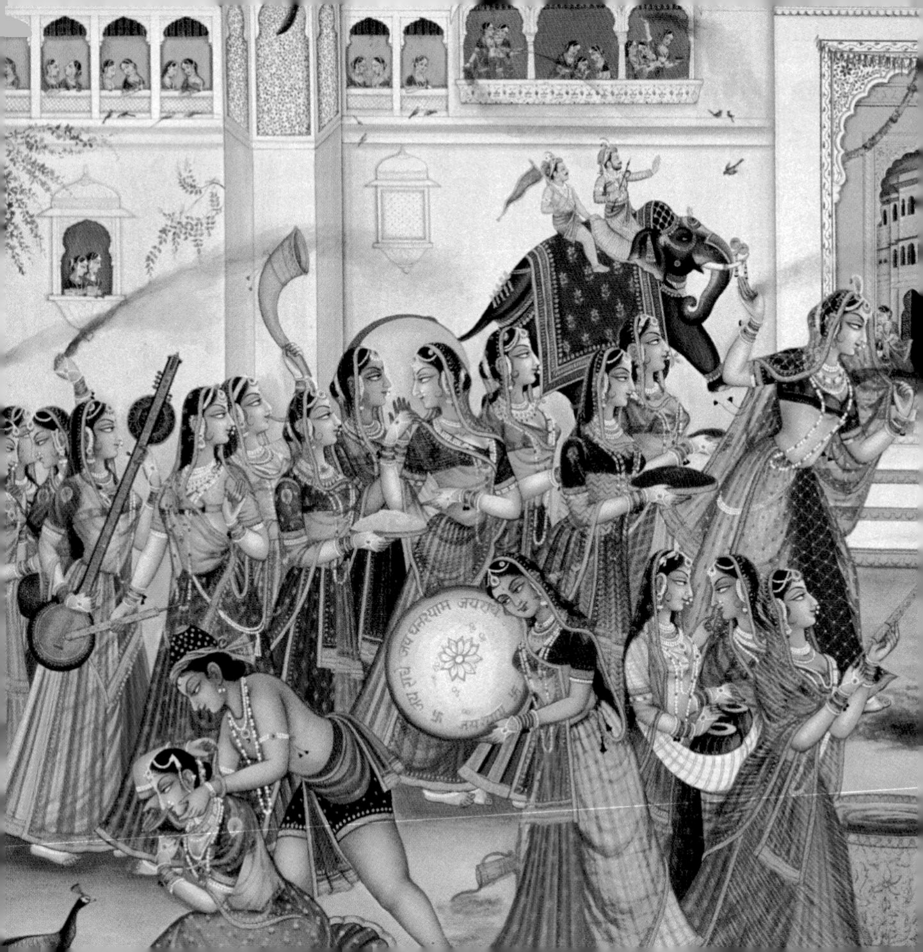
जय राधे जय घनश्याम

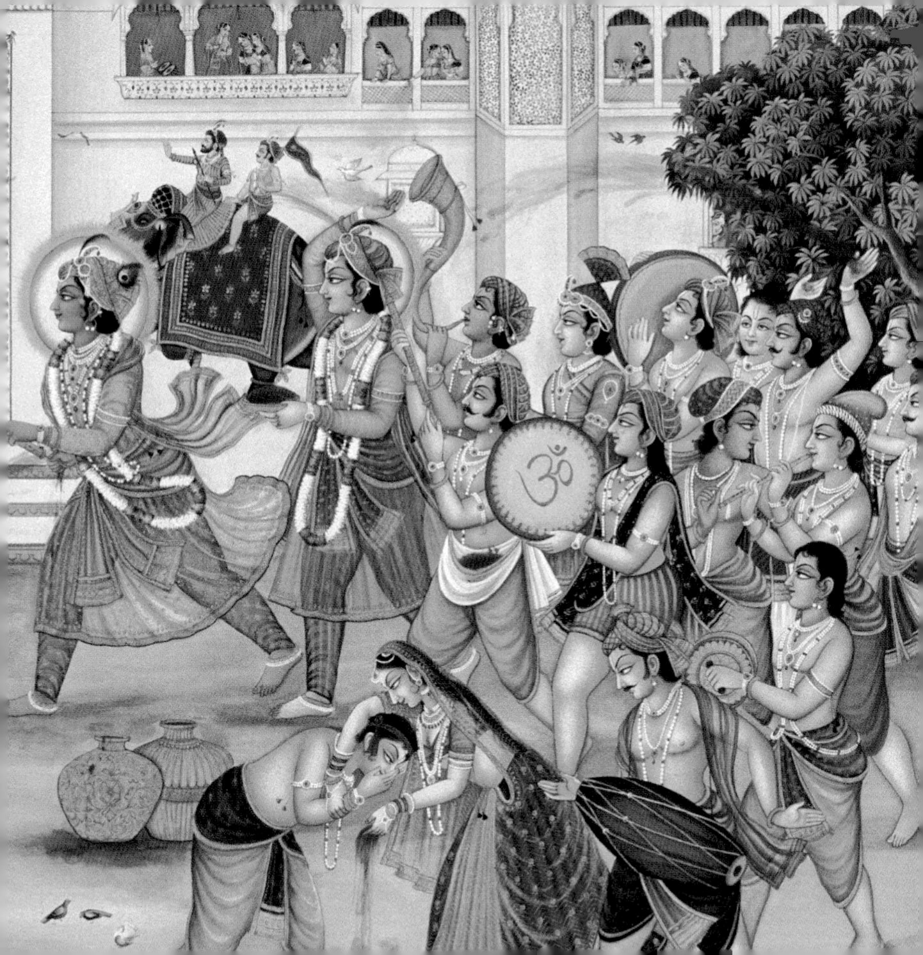

~ Bhoga-ārati ~

by Srila Bhaktivinode Thakur

one

bhaja bhakata-vatsala śrī-gaurahari
śrī-gaurahari sohi goṣṭha-bihārī
nanda-yaśomatī-citta-hārī

two

belā holo, dāmodara, āiso ekhona
bhoga-mandire bosi' koroho bhojana

three

nandera nideśe boise giri-bara-dhārī
baladeva-saha sakhā boise sāri sāri

four

śuktā-śākādi bhāji nālitā kuṣmāṇḍa
ḍāli ḍālnā dugdha-tumbī dadhi mocā-ghaṇṭa

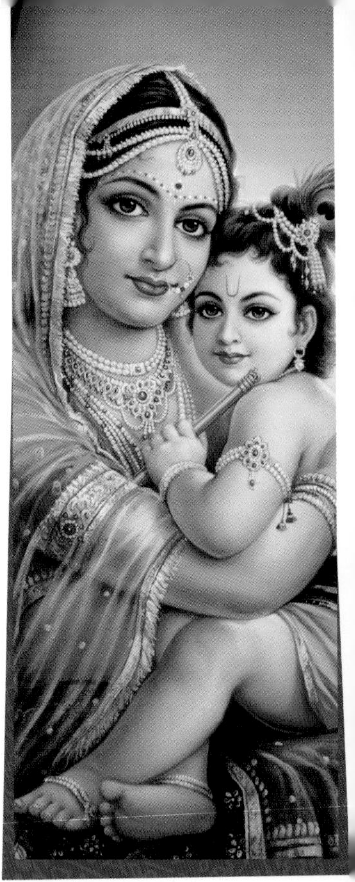

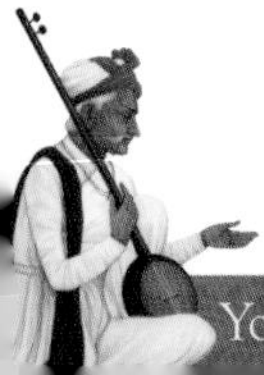

five

mudga-borā māṣa-borā roṭikā ghṛtānna
śaṣkulī piṣṭaka khīra-puli pāyasānna

six

karpūra amṛta-keli rambhā khīra-sāra
amṛta rasālā, amla dvādaśa prakāra

seven

luci-cini sarpurī lāḍḍu rasābolī
bhojana korena kṛṣṇa hoye kutūhalī

eight

rādhikāra pakva anna vividha byañjana
parama ānande kṛṣṇa korena bhojana

nine

chale-bale lāḍḍu khāy śrī-madhumaṅgala
bagala bājāy āra deya hari-bolo

ten

rādhikādi gaṇe heri' nayanera koṇe
tṛpta hoye khāy kṛṣṇa yaśodā-bhavane

eleven

bhojanānte piye kṛṣṇa subāsita bāri
sabe mukha prakṣāloy hoye sāri sāri

twelve

hasta-mukha prakṣāliyā joto sakhā-gaṇe
ānande viśrāma kore baladeva sane

thirteen

jāmbula rasāla āne tāmbūla-masālā
tāhā kheye kṛṣṇa-candra sukhe nidrā gelā

fourteen

viśālākṣa śikhi-puccha cāmara ḍhulāya
apūrba śayyāya kṛṣṇa sukhe nidrā jāya

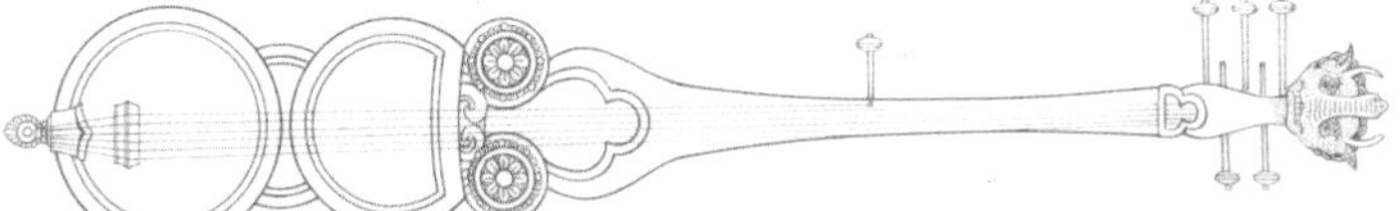

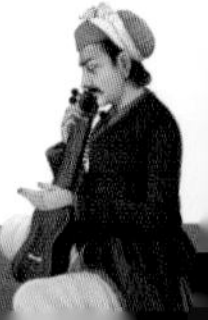

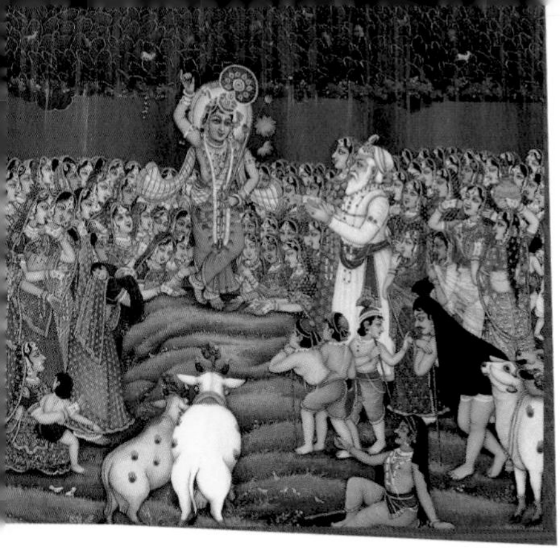

fifteen

yaśomatī-ājñā peye dhaniṣṭhā-ānīto
śrī-kṛṣṇa-prasāda rādhā bhuñje hoye prīto

sixteen

lalitādi-sakhī-gaṇa avaśeṣa pāya
mone mone sukhe rādhā-kṛṣṇa-guṇa gāya

seventeen

hari-līlā eka-mātra jāhāra pramoda
bhogārati gāy ṭhākura bhakativinoda

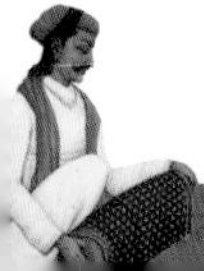

one

Worship Sri Gaurahari, the golden Lord, who is ever affectionate to His devotees. Sri Gaurahari is non-different from Krishna, who sported in the cowherd pastures of Vraja and stole the hearts of Nanda and Yashoda.

two

Mother Yashoda calls out to Krishna: "O Damodar, it has become very late. Come here right now, sit down in the dining hall, and take Your lunch."

three

Directed by Nanda Maharaj, the lifter of Govardhan hill takes His place, after which Baladev and all the cowherd boys sit down in rows.

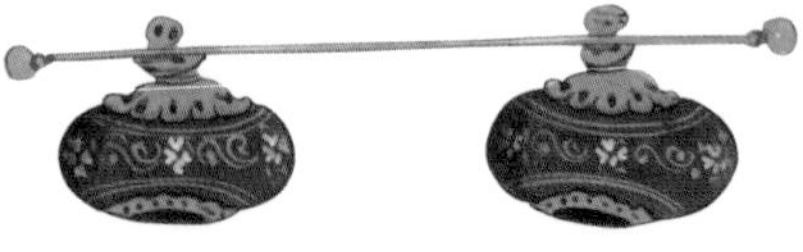

four

They are served a feast of bitter curry and various kinds of spinach, fried delicacies, a salad made of green jute leaves, pumpkin, baskets of fruits, thick yogurt, squash cooked in milk, and vegetable preparations made from the flower of the banana tree.

five

They are also served fried mung dahl patties and urad dahl patties, chapatis, rice with ghee, milksweets, rice flour cakes, thick cooked-down milk, cakes floating in milk, and sweet rice.

six

There is also sweet rice that tastes just like nectar due to its being mixed with camphor. There are bananas, and cheese that is nectarean and delicious. They are also served fruit juices and twelve kinds of sour preparations.

seven

There are puris filled with cream and sugar, laddus and other sweetballs. Krishna eats everything with great delight.

eight

Krishna eats the rice and various curried vegetables cooked by Srimati Radharani in great ecstasy and joy.

nine

Krishna's funny brahmin friend Madhumangal, who is very fond of laddus, gets them by hook or by crook. Eating the laddus, he shouts, "Haribol! Haribol! Give me more!" and makes funny sounds (by slapping his sides under his armpits with his hands).

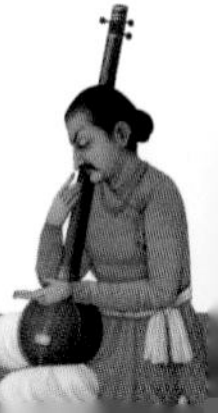

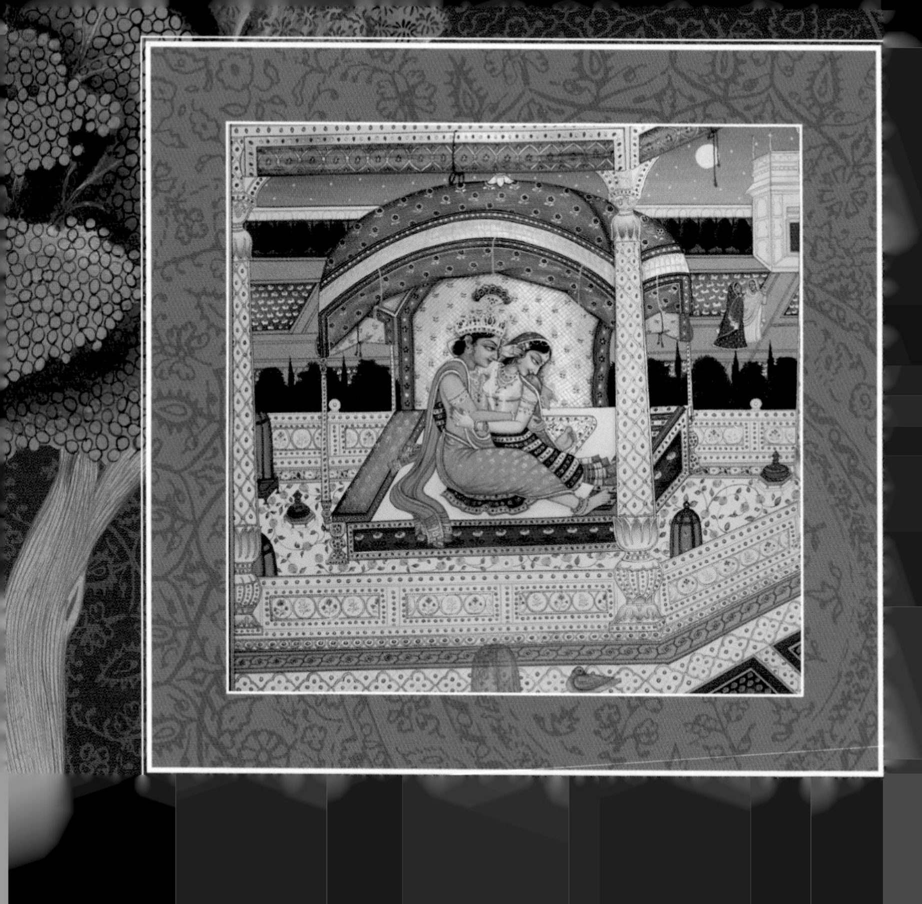

ten

Beholding Radharani and her girlfriends out of the corners of His eyes, Krishna eats His lunch at the house of mother Yashoda with great delight.

eleven

After lunch, Krishna drinks rose-scented water. Then all of the boys stand in line to wash their mouths.

twelve

After washing their mouths, all the cowherd boys take rest along with Lord Balaram, being full of bliss.

thirteen

The two cowherd boys Jambula and Rasala then bring Krishna spiced betel nuts. After eating them, Krishnachandra happily goes to sleep.

fourteen

While Vishalaksha cools Krishna with a fan of peacock feathers, He happily takes rest on an excellent bedstead.

fifteen

At mother Yashoda's request, the gopi Dhanishtha brings the remnants of food left on Krishna's plate to Srimati Radharani, who eats them with great delight.

sixteen

Lalita and the cowherd girls receive Radha's remnants. Then with great joy, they sing the glories of Radha and Krishna within their hearts.

seventeen

Thakur Bhaktivinode, whose one and only joy is the pastimes of Lord Hari, sings this bhoga arati song.

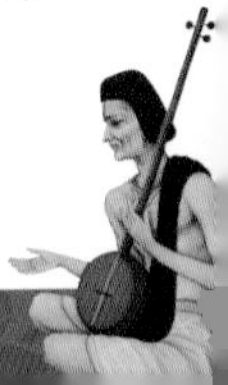

~ Śrī Rādhikā-stava ~

"Glorifying Radha"
by Srila Rupa Goswami

refrain

rādhe jaya jaya mādhava-dayite
gokula-taruṇī-maṇḍala-mahite

one

dāmodara-rati-vardhana-veśe
hari-niṣkuṭa-vṛndā-vipineśe

two

vṛṣabhānūdadhi-nava-śaśi-lekhe
lalitā-sakhi guṇa-ramita-viśākhe

three

karuṇāṁ kuru mayi karuṇā-bharite
sanaka-sanātana-varṇita-carite

refrain

O Radha! All glories to You, beloved of Madhava. You are worshiped by all the young girls of Gokul.

one

You dress Yourself in such a way as to increase Lord Damodar's love for and attachment to You. You are the queen of Lord Hari's pleasure grove, Vrindavan.

two

O new moon who has arisen from the ocean of King Vrishabhanu. O friend of Lalita! O You who enchant Vishakha by Your wonderful qualities.

three

O You who are filled with compassion. You whose divine characteristics are described by the great sages Sanaka and Sanatan. O Radha! Please be merciful to me.

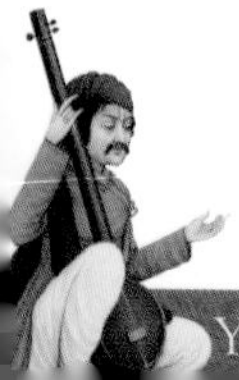

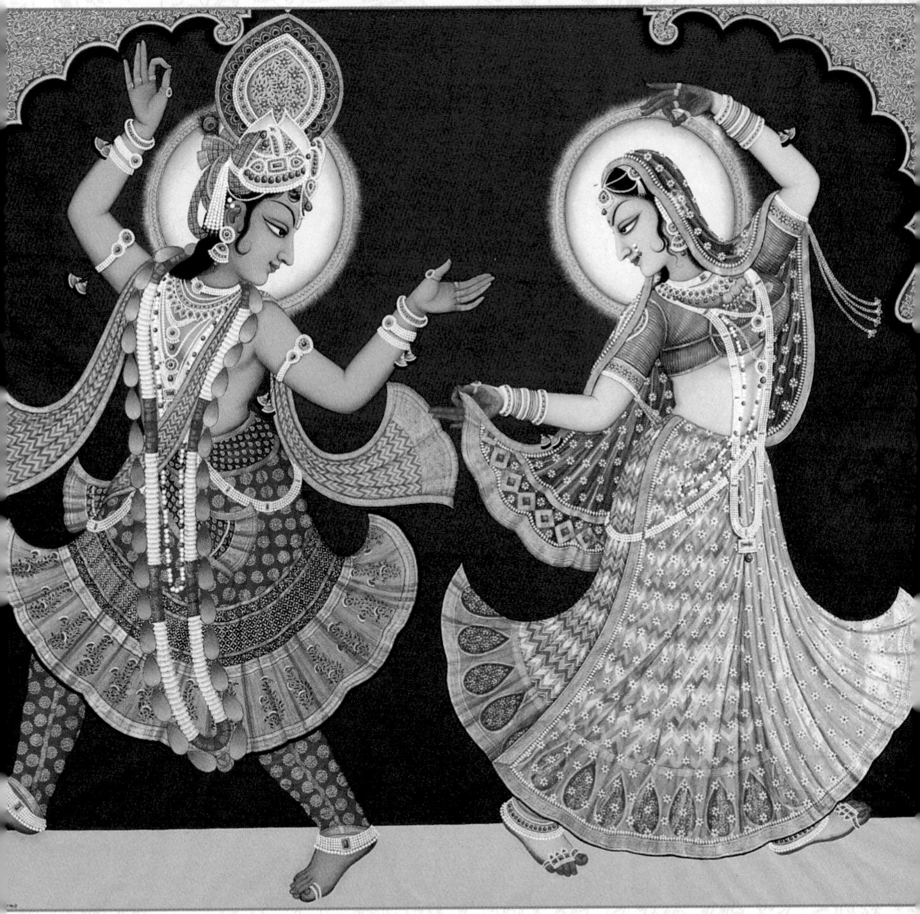

~ Vaiṣṇava Vijñapti ~

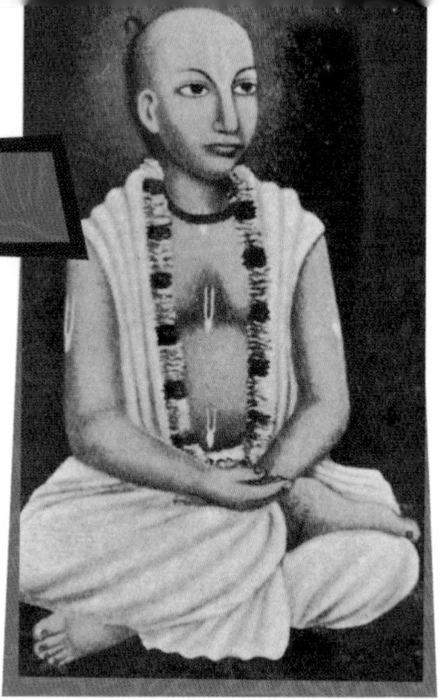

"Prayer to the Vaishnava"
by Srila Narottam Das Thakur

one

ei bāro karuṇā koro vaiṣṇava-gosāñi
patita-pāvana tomā bine keho nāi

two

jāhāra nikaṭe gele pāpa dūre jāy
emona doyāla prabhu kebā kothā pāy

three

gaṅgāra paraśa hoile paścāte pāvan
darśane pavitra koro - ei tomāra guṇ

four

hari-sthāne aparādhe tāre hari-nām
tomā-sthāne aparādhe nāhi paritrāṇ

five

tomāra hṛdoye sadā govinda-viśrām
govinda kohena - mora vaiṣṇava parāṇ

six

prati-janme kori āśā caraṇera dhūli
narottame koro doyā āpanāra boli'

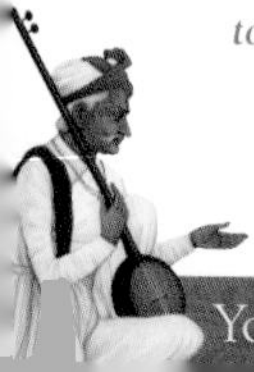

one

O Vaishnava Goswami, please be merciful to me now. There is no one except you who can rescue the fallen souls.

two

Where does anyone get such a merciful master, by whose mere presence all sins go far away?

three

After bathing in the waters of the sacred Ganges many times, one becomes purified, but just by the sight of you, the fallen souls are purified. This is your divine quality.

four

The Holy Name delivers one from offences committed against the Lord, but it does not pardon offences that are committed against you, O Vaishnava Thakur.

five

Your heart is always the resting place of Lord Govinda, and Lord Govinda says, "The Vaishnavas are in My heart."

six

I desire to obtain the dust of Your holy feet in every birth I may take. Please consider Narottam Yours, and be merciful to him.

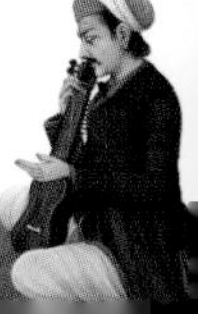

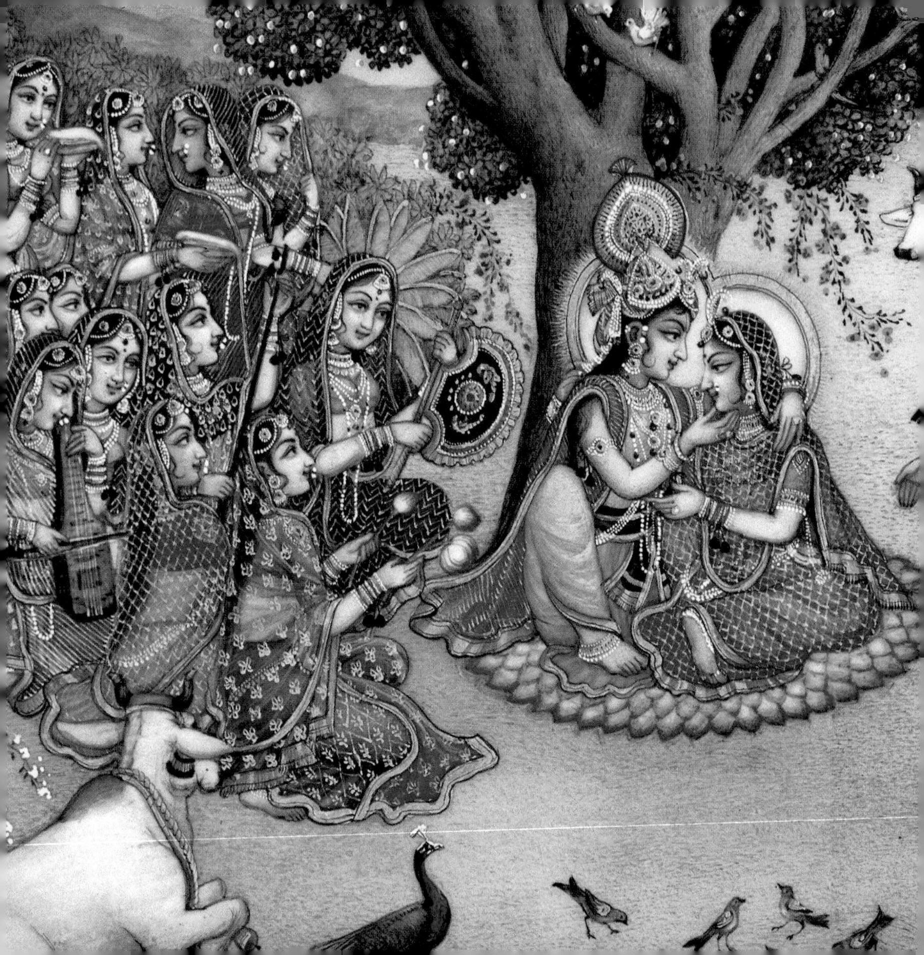

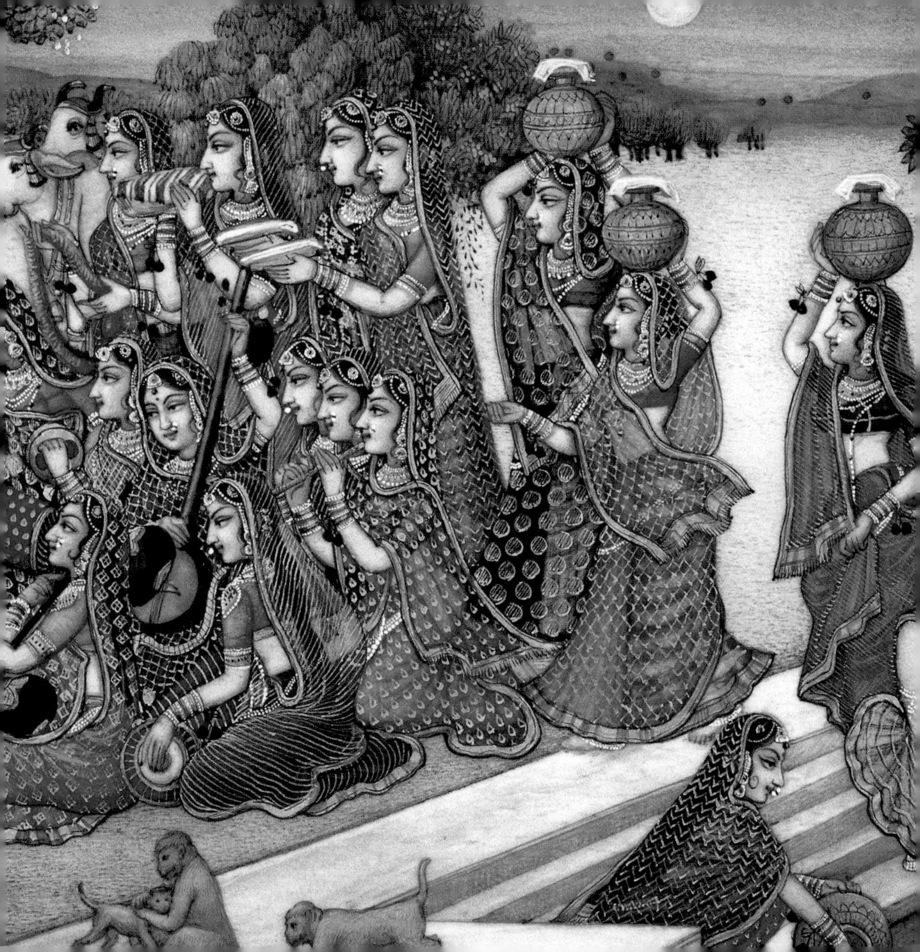

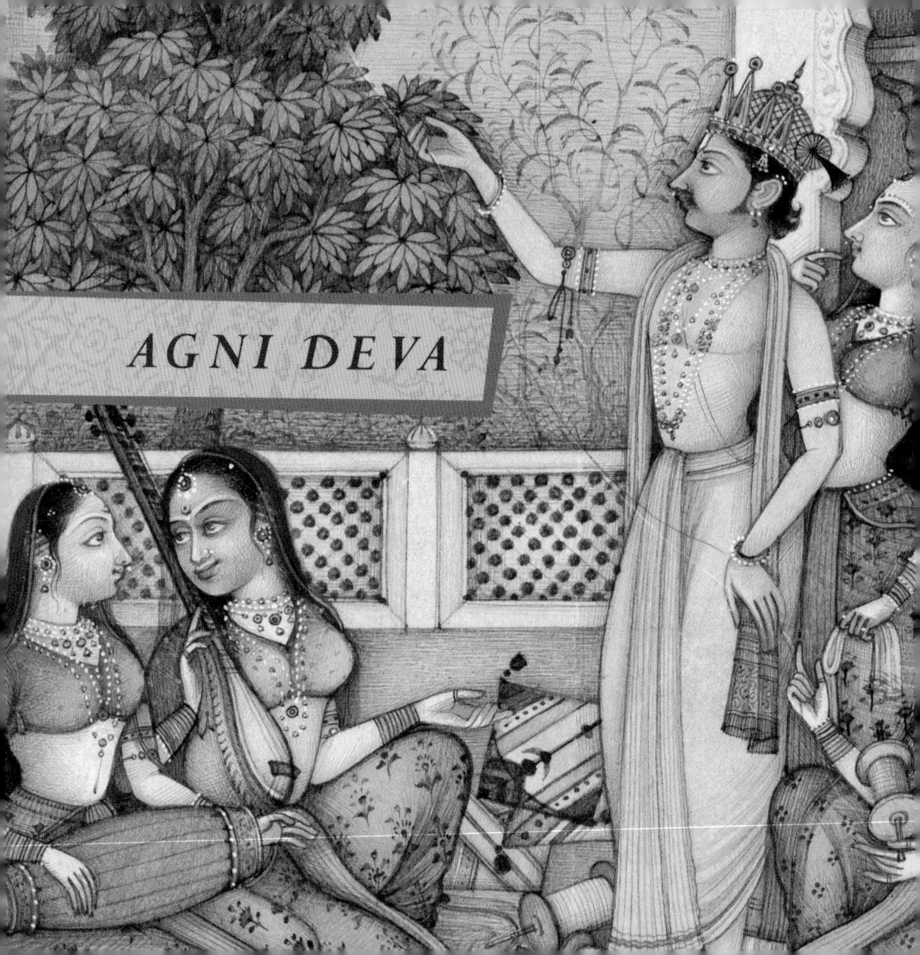
AGNI DEVA

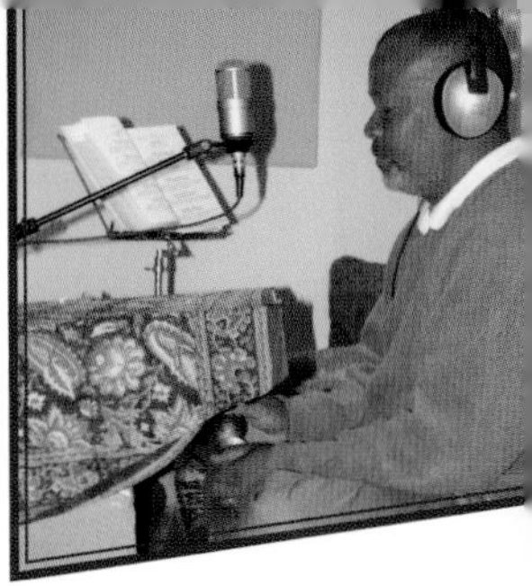

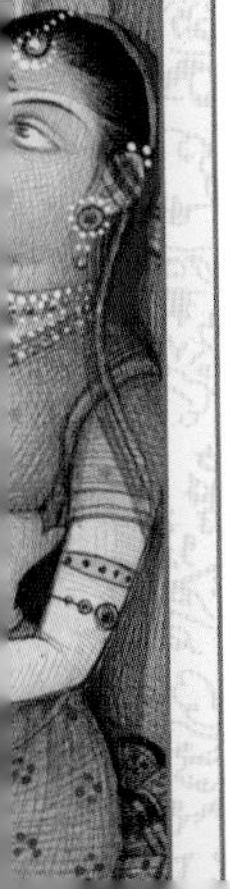

Agni Deva was born in Trinidad, West Indies, and moved to New York in his youth. His study of Vedic philosophy led him to discover the devotional music of West Bengal. In 1972 he began publicly performing *bhajan* and *kirtan* in the traditional Bengali style. He later toured with the South Asian Cultural Exhibition, singing on university campuses throughout the United States. In his numerous trips to India he has sought out master *kirtaniyas* who have helped him evolve a truly traditional style. His influences include the work of A.C. Bhaktivedanta Swami Prabhupada, from whom he received mantra initiation into the path of pure devotion following Sri Chaitanya. Along with his musical and spiritual pursuits, Agni Deva's other passion is cooking. He owns and operates Govinda's Vegetarian Buffet in Santa Rosa, California.

Kirtan is the sixth recording from Agni Deva, along with *Bhakti Rasa*, *Tribute to Prabhupada*, *Treasure of the Holy Name*, and *Live in New Dwarka*. It is the second in the Mandala trilogy, along with *Smaranam* and his upcoming release *Waves of Bhakti*.

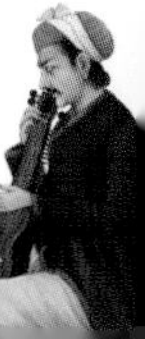

INSTRUMENTS

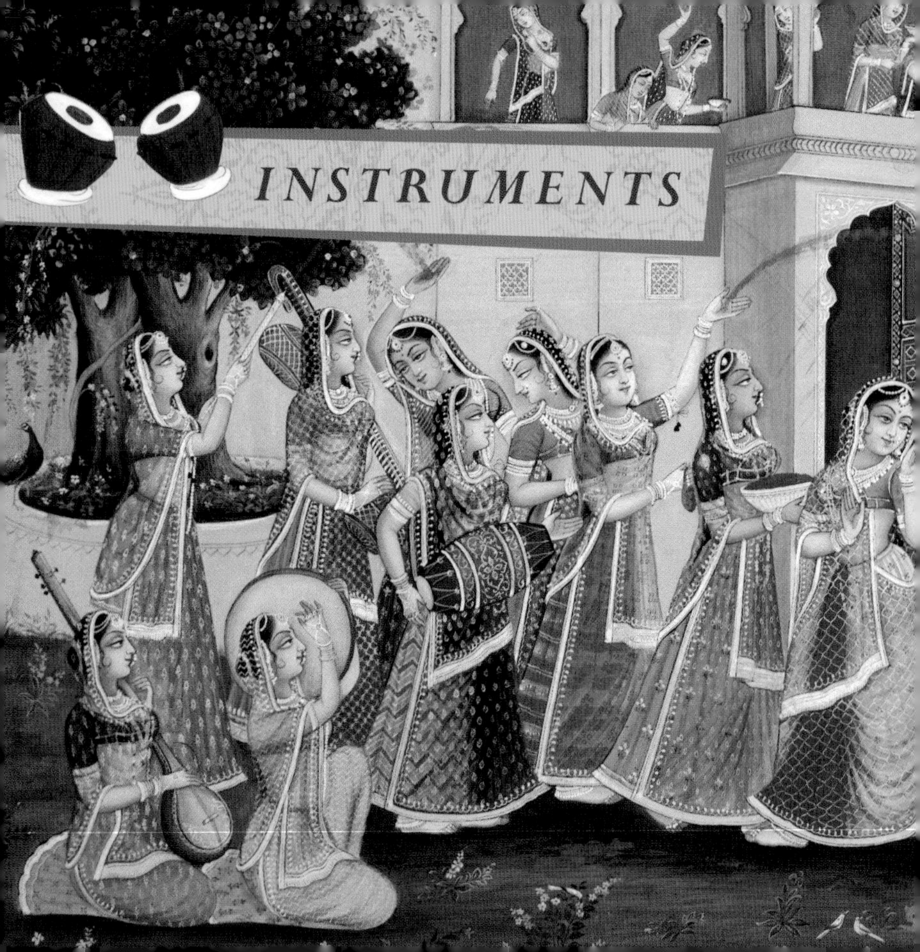

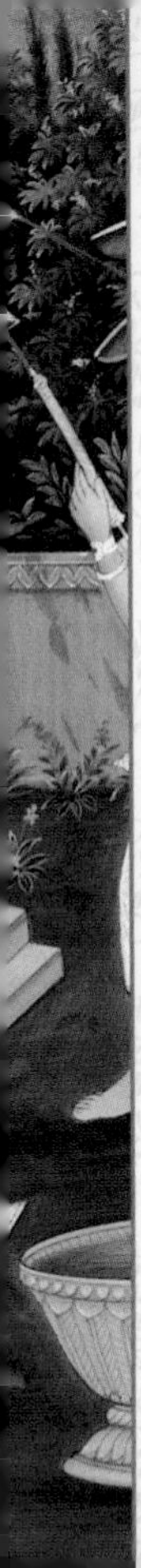

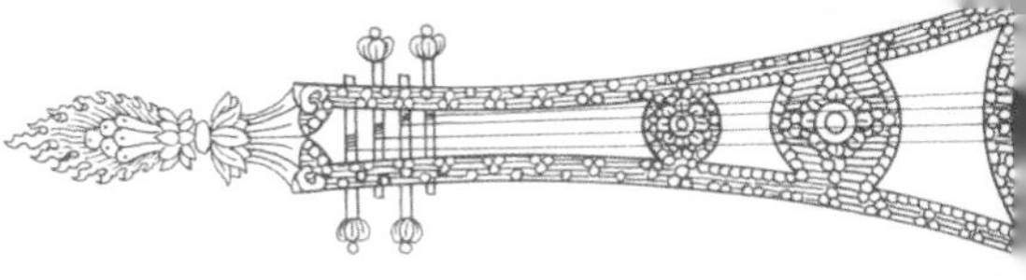

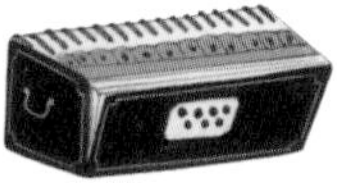

The Harmonium—The harmonium is a Western instrument that originated in Germany and England and became popular among immigrant pioneers in the American West in the nineteenth century. Around the same time, the British brought the harmonium to India, where it was quickly absorbed into the Indian music culture. Although not a traditional Indian instrument, it was admired for its portability and drone quality, which made it uniquely appropriate to the Indian aesthetic.

The Cello—The cello was first made in its current shape in the mid-1600s. Its predecessor was the viola da gamba (Italian for knee fiddle), which had six or seven strings and tied frets across its finger board. The current design of the cello allows the artist to play with a more melodic and expressive approach (instead of the viola da gamba's chordal approach), a development consistent with the changes of European music during the seventeenth century.

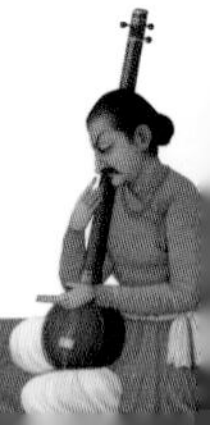

Mridanga—The word *mridanga* is derived from *mrid* "clay" and *anga* "body," meaning that it is an instrument, a drum in this case, whose body or shell is made of clay. According to other sources, it derives from *mridan* and *ga*, meaning "beaten while moving," as its design permits the drum to be hung around the neck and played while walking or even dancing.

This instrument has a unique history connected to the cultural and spiritual evolution of Sri Chaitanya in sixteenth-century Bengal. It is said that Sri Chaitanya ordered his associates to construct clay drums instead of heavy and costly wooden drums.

A number of styles of mridanga playing developed known as Manoharshayi, Mandarini, and Garanhati. These schools trace their lineages back to Srinivas Acharya, Shyamananda Pandit, and Narottam Das Thakur, respectively. Although these ancient traditions have undergone change and are little practiced in their original form, the mridanga continues to be popular in Vaishnava sacred music.

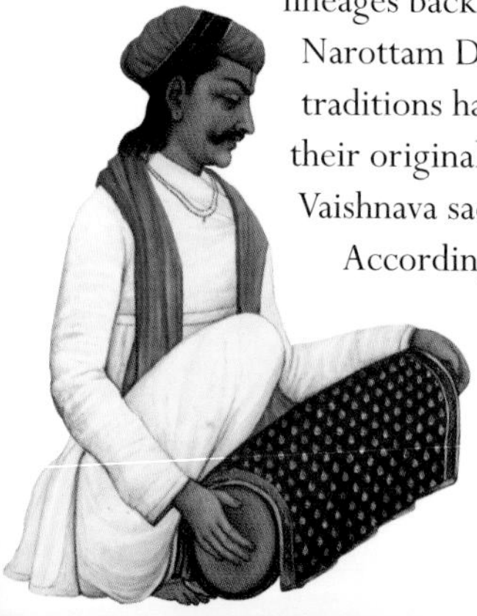

According to the Manoharshayi school, Lord Krishna's flute pleaded with him not to be left behind when he became incarnate as Sri Chaitanya. Krishna thus allowed the flute to accompany him in his advent as Sri Chaitanya in the mridanga form.

It is also said that Sri Chaitanya prayed to Lord Jagannath for the mantras with which to play the mridanga, and the revelation of these mantras was given to Gadadhar Pandit, who became the first player of this divine instrument.

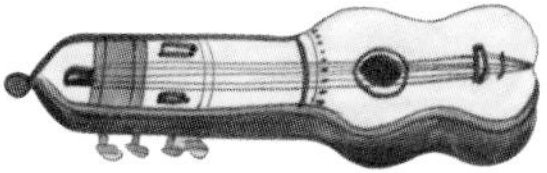

Sarangi—The sarangi is a bowed Indian fiddle with a goatskin top that is played with the cuticles of the left hand. It has three main strings and thirty-six resonating strings that are grouped into four different tuned sets. Unlike the sitar or sarod, which were played at the courts of medieval Indian nobility, the sarangi is considered to be a folklore instrument that was primarily used to accompany singers. Its popularity declined as the aforementioned instruments gained more and more recognition. The instrument used on this recording was built by Ricki Ram in Dehli and modified by Hans Christian.

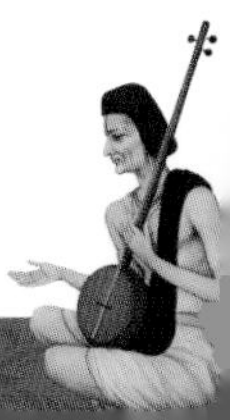

NYCKELHARPA—The nyckelharpa is a bowed Scandinavian key fiddle, with four main strings and twelve resonating strings. The player pushes a set of wooden keys that in turn press against the strings. Its origins extend back to the Middle Ages.

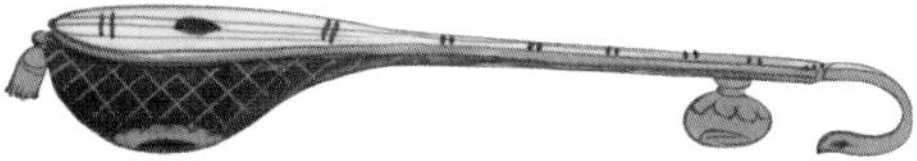

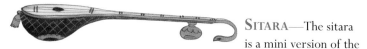

SITARA—The sitara is a mini version of the Indian sitar with curved brass frets, four play strings, eight resonating strings, and two arched bridges that create the characteristic buzzing sound. The particular instrument played by Hans is custom made from solid ebony by a San Francisco Bay Area instrument maker.

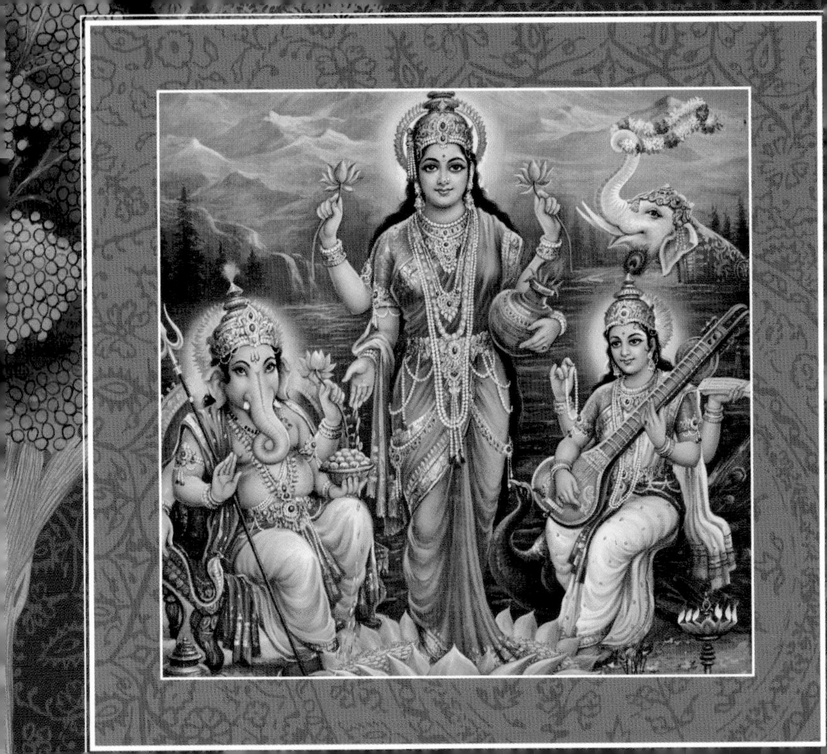

Bibliography

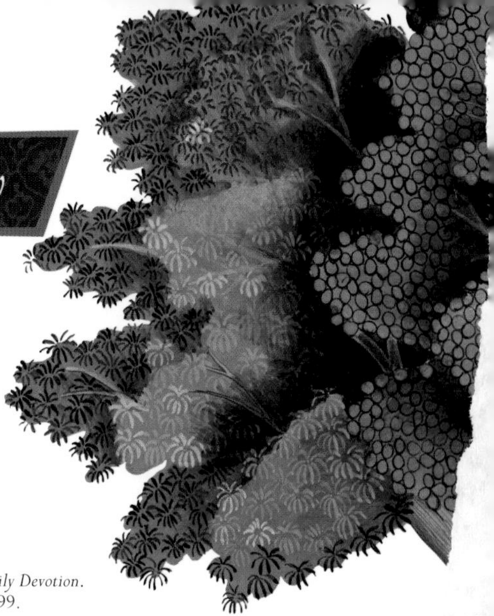

Beevers, John. *The Autobiography of St. Therese of Lisieux: The Story of a Soul*. New York: Doubleday & Company, 1957.

Brown, Daniel P., Jack Engler, and Ken Wilber. *Transformations of Consciousness: Convention and Contemplative Perspectives on Development*. Boston: Shambala, 1998.

Das, Raghava Chaitanya. *Divine Name*. Chandigarh: HKT, 1998.

Maslow, Abrahan H. *Religions, Values, and Peak-experiences*. New York: The Viking Press, 1974.

Puri, Swami B. P. *Art of Sadhana: A Guide to Daily Devotion*. San Francisco: Mandala Publishing Group, 1999.

Sridhar, Bhakti Raksaka. *The Golden Volcano of Divine Love*. San Jose: Guardian of Devotion Press, 1984.

Swami, A. C. Bhaktivedanta. *The Golden Avatar*. Philippines: Bhaktivedanta Book Trust, 1981.

Wilber, Ken. *Sex, Ecology, and Spirituality: The Spirit of Evolution*. Boston: Shambala, 1995.

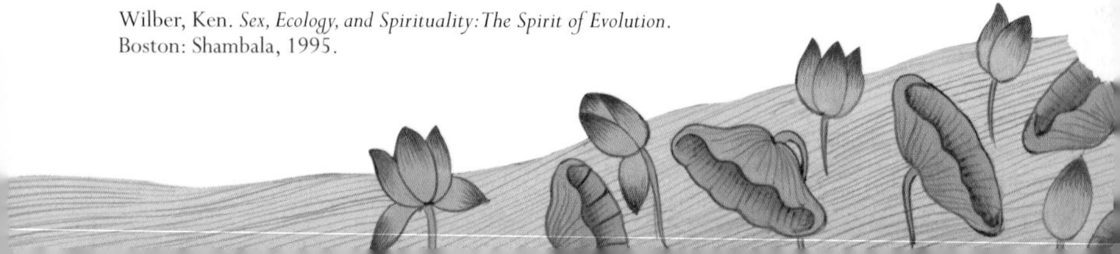

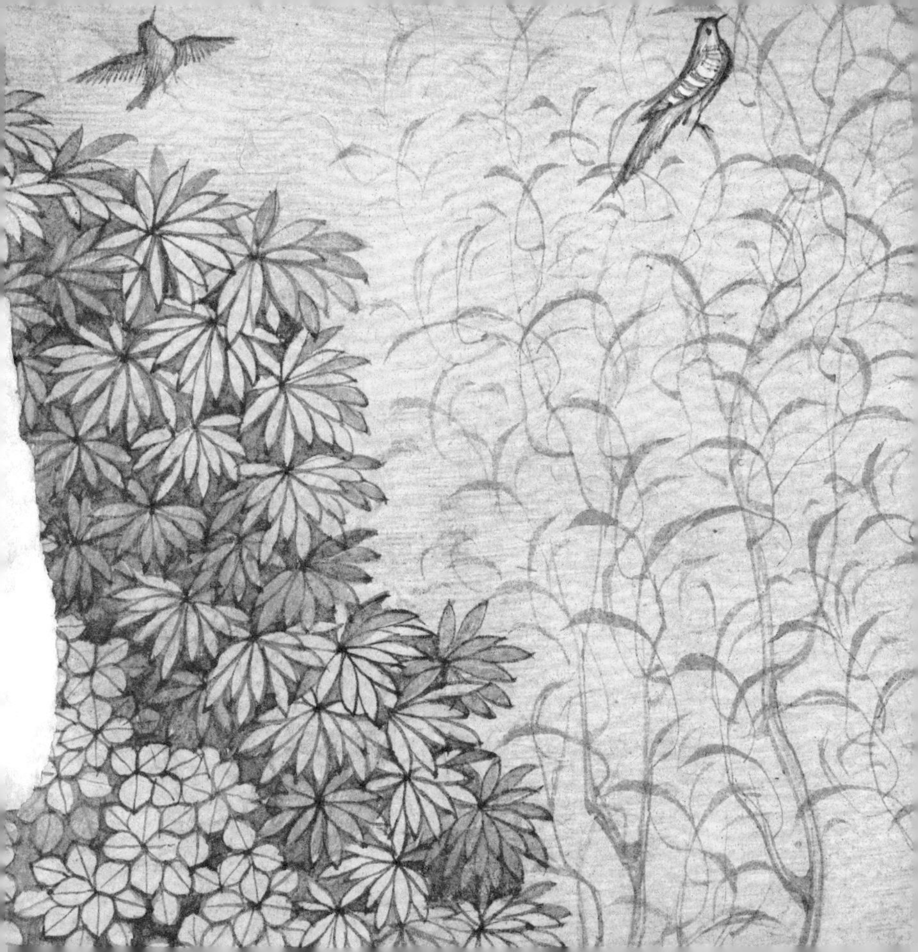

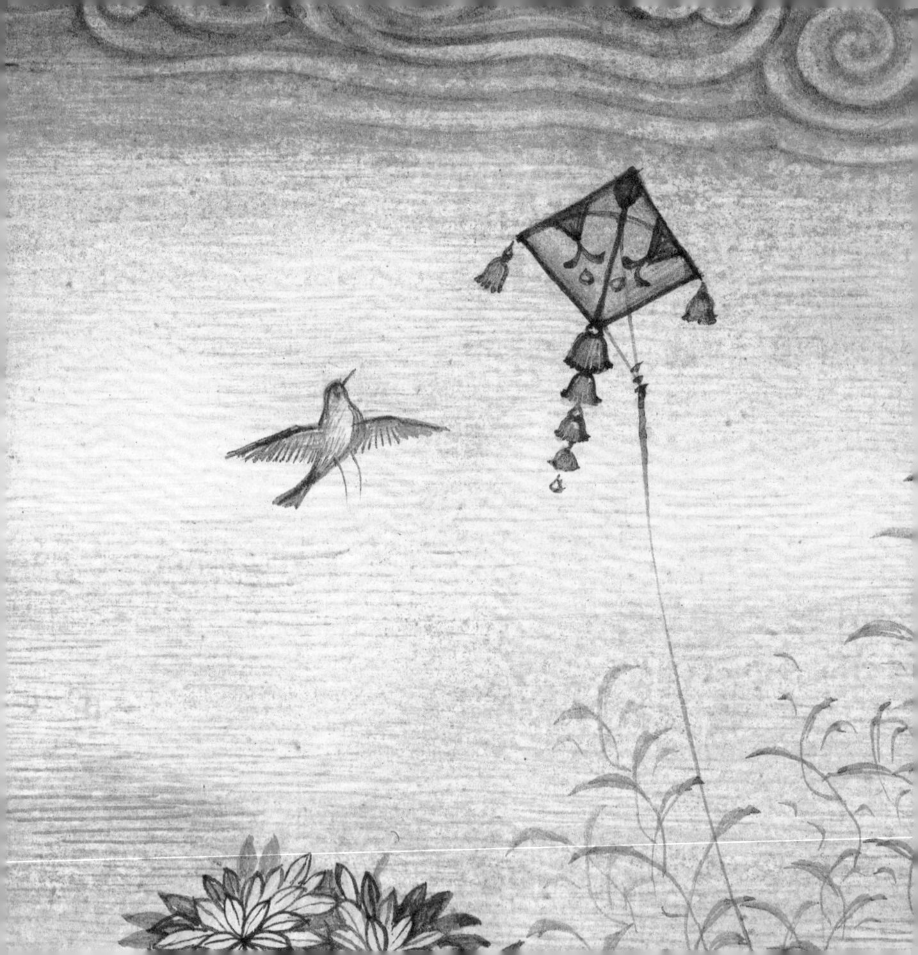